LEADER/ACTIVITY
GUIDE

A Hands-On Guide Filled With Delicious Learning!

A Companion to

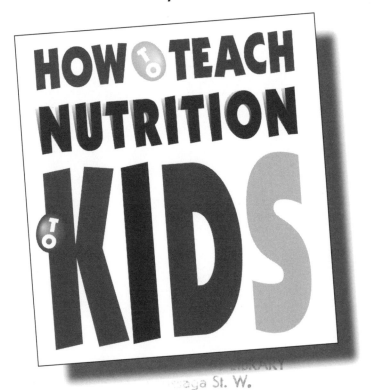

HOW TO TEACH NUTRITION TO KIDS

Connie Liakos Evers, M.S., R.D. & Hugh-Man Bean, R.B.
(Registered Beanologist)

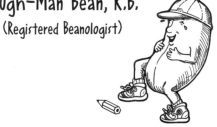

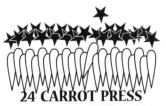

24 CARROT PRESS

DONATED BY:
THE SIMCOE COUNTY
DIABETES PREVENTION PROJECT

Cover, Design, & Illustration: Carol Buckle Design + Illustration
Typesetting: William H. Brunson, Typography Services

Printed in the United States of America

ISBN 0-9647970-6-2

Published by

24 CARROT PRESS

P.O. Box 23546
Tigard, OR 97281-3546
503-524-9318
eversc@teleport.com
http://www.nutritionforkids.com

Table of Contents

Introduction

Since the publication of *How to Teach Nutrition to Kids*, I have received many requests for an accompanying leader/activity guide. Readers have asked for a guide that includes copy-ready masters with fun, easy-to-use activities. Many have also asked for ways to evaluate student progress at making healthful dietary changes.

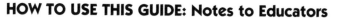

"Attention please! This is important, useful stuff that you need to know"

I am happy to say that here it is! I have assembled many of the activities that I commonly use when I teach elementary-aged children, including 27 new lessons that are unique to this guide.

Before you dive right into the activity sections, please read the recommendations below on how to use this guide.

By the way, that little guy that just popped up is my good friend, Hugh-Man Bean. Hugh is here primarily for the children who will be using the activity sheets but you may see him around in other places. Please humor him. He is only Hugh-man, after all!

HOW TO USE THIS GUIDE: Notes to Educators

This leader/activity guide is designed to be used in conjunction with the book *How to Teach Nutrition to Kids*, which includes background information about nutrition, tips on how to promote positive food messages, the importance of making nutrition fun, integrated, and behavior focused, and more than 200 activities to help you implement these concepts. Ordering information for this book is listed on the last page of this guide.

This guide can be used in the following ways:

▪ As you are planning your nutrition and health curriculum, this guide will provide you with structure and hands-on activities. The suggestions for evaluation will help you to assess students' progress in adopting healthful eating and exercise behaviors.

▪ Many of the lesson ideas in this guide work well as "stand alone" activities that you can teach throughout the year as a reinforcement for healthful eating and as a way to integrate nutrition concepts into your curriculum. For example, in chapter two students learn the importance of goal setting, a skill which transfers to study habits and other areas of life. In chapter three, they explore advertising from a food point-of-view, which fits well with a general study of advertising.

▪ This guide also provides many ideas for food and nutrition lessons that can be used during special events and celebrations such as wellness week, National Nutrition Month, National School Lunch Week, heart month and health fairs.

THE P.I.E. SYSTEM

The P.I.E. system was introduced in the index of *How to Teach Nutrition to Kids*. The activity codes are defined below:

P Primary Level: Kindergarten–Second Grade

I Intermediate Level: Third–Sixth Grades

E Either Level: Activities are adaptable for all ages.

These are not carved-in-stone levels, but simply guidelines to help you when planning lessons. You will find that many of the activities reach beyond these age ranges and may be adaptable for early childhood or the middle school grade levels.

Look for one of the letters in the left-hand corner of each activity page that lets you know at a glance the intended grade level.

EVALUATION

A common question among nutrition educators is, "How do I know that I am making a difference?" Oftentimes, children (adults too!) may learn a great deal about food and nutrition but fail to put their knowledge into practice.

Throughout this guide, there will be suggestions on how to assess the changes in nutrition knowledge and behavior of the children you teach. The self-assessment activities in chapter 1 provide the cornerstone for evaluating the children's progress.

NOTES TO PARENTS

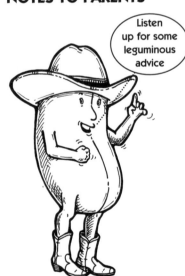

Listen up for some leguminous advice

If you are serious about getting your kids to eat right, there are a few "beans" of wisdom that you need to know. These are common sense guidelines, yet they make all the difference in helping your children form healthful, lifelong eating habits.

■ Be a role model for healthful eating. Children really do learn best by example.

■ Make family meals a priority. Not only do children form better food habits, it is also a great opportunity for family communication.

■ Buy *mostly* healthy foods that follow the tenet of the Food Guide Pyramid. There's nothing wrong with occasional treats and sweets, but the core of the diet should consist of whole grains, fruits, vegetables, lean protein foods, and low-fat dairy products.

■ Monitor television, videos, and computer time. Encourage a balance of activities, including plenty of time for good ol' outside play!

WHAT KIDS NEED TO KNOW*

Emphasize food as it relates to life today.

You will lose kids' attention faster than they can say "osteoporosis" if too much emphasis is placed on how proper nutrition prevents disease. If you succeed in reaching them with the good nutrition message today, their tomorrows will likely be healthier too.

Remind children that healthful food promotes achievement. In school or on the playing field, kids who eat well perform better and achieve higher levels of mastery. A nutritious diet fuels the body for learning, growth, sports, and play.

Well-nourished kids look better, too! Children who eat a balanced diet have bright, sparkly eyes, healthy skin, hair, and teeth, and bodies that look and feel great.

The message of good nutrition is summed up in the first six *Dietary Guidelines for Americans*.

Adults and kids over the age of two are advised to eat from a wide selection of foods, emphasize grains, fruits and vegetables, moderate the amount of fat, sugar, and sodium they eat, and keep their weight in check. Simple advice that's often hard to put into practice!

Two important practical tools for meeting these guidelines are the *Food Guide Pyramid* and the *Nutrition Facts* food label. A "picture" of what a healthful diet looks like, the pyramid is especially useful as a teaching aid for children. The revised food label is a simplified, yet effective, device for analyzing foods and comparing their nutrient content.

Teach children to refuel their bodies!

Because of their smaller stomach capacity and tremendous energy needs, kids require frequent meals and snacks. Behavior problems at times are merely the result of an empty stomach.

Somehow, "snacking" has taken on a negative connotation in our society, perhaps because it is often linked with low-nutrient foods. Done right, snacks can and do make a big contribution to daily nutrition. Healthful snacks should mirror meals—emphasizing healthful foods, but in smaller quantities.

Breakfast is the meal most directly connected to school achievement. Kids who skip breakfast have shorter attention spans, do poorly in tasks requiring concentration, and even score lower on standard achievement tests.

Young bodies need to move!

Nutrition studies show that the increasing problem of childhood obesity stems more from inactivity than overeating. An intricate balance exists between food and physical activity. A nutrition unit will be decidedly lacking if it fails to present the exercise part of the equation. Kids enjoy learning about nutrition when it is presented from a fitness perspective. Physical fitness should also be part of the daily classroom routine, especially in schools that limit PE to once or twice weekly.

Teach children to critically analyze the influences of the media.

If children are to resist the allure of the media, advertisements, and other societal influences, they must learn to identify the intent of the messages.

*Adapted from *How to Teach Nutrition to Kids*, pages 23–26

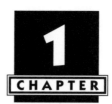

CHAPTER

Self Assessment

NOTES TO EDUCATORS

The activities in this chapter form the basis of evaluating the effectiveness of your nutrition education unit.

■ Begin your nutrition unit by having the children track their eating and exercise habits using one or more of the methods outlined in this chapter. Children have *three* options for tracking their daily eating habits, including the **personal pyramid**, **pocket tally** or the **nutrition abacus**.

The serving size activities will help children better gauge the number of servings that they are actually eating, a difficult concept for people of all ages!

■ Encourage children to complete their **Weekly Activity Check-off** each day. Stress the important relationship between food and activity and how an increase in activity requires an increase in fuel (food!).

■ Today's children are becoming increasingly obsessed about their body shape and size, developing unhealthy attitudes that may lead to disordered eating (for a discussion of this issue, please see pages 20–26 in *How to Teach Nutrition to Kids*). The **My Body is a Great Body!** activity sheet is designed to help children identify their strengths and contribute to a more healthy body image. In conjunction with this activity, discuss how bodies come in a wide variety of shapes and sizes and that everyone grows and develops at different rates.

■ Throughout the nutrition unit, students should continue to monitor and track their progress. As they learn more about nutrition and fitness and set goals for their personal health, these self-monitoring activities will allow them to visually chart their progress over time.

■ During the school year, children should periodically be encouraged to reassess their food and activity behaviors.

■ This is also a great homework activity that can involve the entire family in assessing diet and activity patterns.

■ Teachers and adult leaders will also benefit from tracking eating and exercise habits. Setting a good example is a powerful reinforcer for children.

SIZING UP MY DIET

🅴 Personal Pyramid

NAME _____

DIRECTIONS:

Each time you eat or drink anything, draw or write the name of the food or beverage in the correct food group space on the pyramid. If you eat a food such as cheese pizza, you will record the crust in the grain group, the sauce in the vegetable group and the cheese in the dairy group.

The *Serving Guidelines* charts on page 16 will help if you have questions about where to put foods on your personal pyramid.

At the end of the day, answer the questions at the bottom of this page.

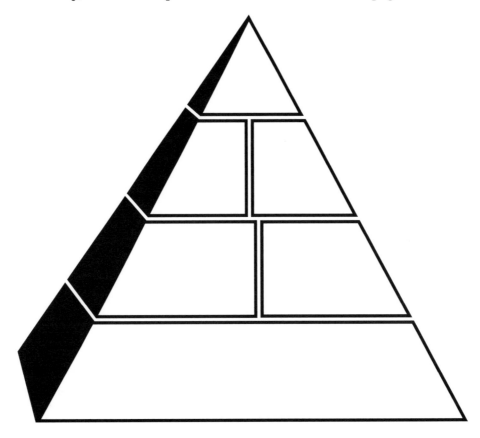

Questions

1. Check your record for balance:

   Did you eat something from every food group?

   List any groups with fewer than the suggested servings.

   List any groups with more than the suggested servings.

2. Was today a "normal" day? Was there anything that happened today that changed your eating habits?

3. Are there changes you could make to better balance your "personal pyramid?"

SIZING UP MY DIET

E Personal Pyramid

NAME _____

DIRECTIONS:

Each time you eat or drink anything, draw or write the name of the food or beverage in the correct food group space on the pyramid. If you eat a food such as cheese pizza, you will record the crust in the grain group, the sauce in the vegetable group and the cheese in the dairy group.

The *Serving Guidelines* charts on page 16 will help if you have questions about where to put foods on your personal pyramid.

At the end of the day, answer the questions at the bottom of this page.

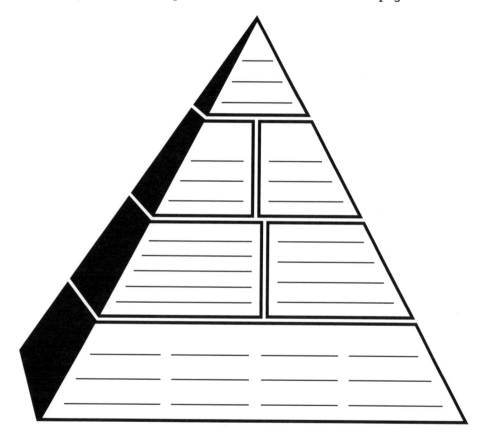

Questions

1. Check your record for balance:

   Did you eat something from every food group?

   List any groups with fewer than the suggested servings.

   List any groups with more than the suggested servings.

2. Was today a "normal" day? Was there anything that happened today that changed your eating habits?

3. Are there changes you could make to better balance your "personal pyramid?"

SIZING UP MY DIET

🅴 Pocket Tally

DIRECTIONS:

1. Cut out the pocket tallies on the next page. Staple together and put in a handy place so you will remember to write down the food you eat.

2. Each time you eat or drink anything, write the name of the food or beverage on your pocket tally. Next, place a tally mark in the correct food group. For example, if you had cereal, yogurt and juice for breakfast, place tally marks in the Grain, Dairy and Fruit groups.

The *Serving Guidelines* charts on page 16 will help you to decide where to place foods in the food group categories.

At the end of each day, answer the questions at the bottom of this page.

SAMPLE:

Name **Alison Kelly**

MY POCKET TALLY

What I Ate Today:	Grains	Fruits	Vegetables	Dairy	Protein	Fats, Oils & Sweets
Breakfast: 1 Bagel / Cream Cheese / 1 Banana / 1 c. 1% Milk	II	I		I		I
Lunch: Turkey Sandwich w/mayo / Carrots & apple / 1 carton 1% Milk	II	I	I	I	I	I
Dinner: 2 slices cheese pizza / 1 serving broccoli / 3 cookies / water	II		I	I		I
Snacks: 10 chewy candies / 1 c. orange juice / 1 peanut butter sandwich	II	I			I	I
Totals:	8	3	2	3	2	4

HOW DID I DO TODAY?

1. Did I eat breakfast?

2. Did I eat the suggested number of servings from each group?

3. Did I make progress on a personal nutrition goal?

Explain _____

_____

12

MY POCKET TALLY

Name _____

What I Ate Today:

	Grains	Fruits	Vegetables	Dairy	Protein	Fats, Oils & Sweets
Breakfast: _____ _____ _____						
Lunch: _____ _____ _____						
Dinner: _____ _____ _____						
Snacks: _____ _____ _____						
Totals:						

MY POCKET TALLY

Name _____

What I Ate Today:

	Grains	Fruits	Vegetables	Dairy	Protein	Fats, Oils & Sweets
Breakfast: _____ _____ _____						
Lunch: _____ _____ _____						
Dinner: _____ _____ _____						
Snacks: _____ _____ _____						
Totals:						

MY POCKET TALLY

Name _____

What I Ate Today:

	Grains	Fruits	Vegetables	Dairy	Protein	Fats, Oils & Sweets
Breakfast: _____ _____ _____						
Lunch: _____ _____ _____						
Dinner: _____ _____ _____						
Snacks: _____ _____ _____						
Totals:						

MY POCKET TALLY

Name _____

What I Ate Today:

	Grains	Fruits	Vegetables	Dairy	Protein	Fats, Oils & Sweets
Breakfast: _____ _____ _____						
Lunch: _____ _____ _____						
Dinner: _____ _____ _____						
Snacks: _____ _____ _____						
Totals:						

SIZING UP MY DIET

E Nutrition Abacus

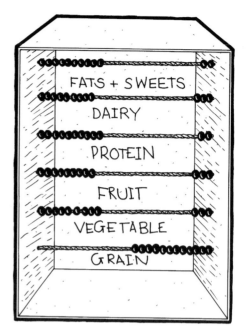

YOU WILL NEED:

shoebox
string or twine
72 buttons or beads (in six different colors, if possible)
markers or crayons

DIRECTIONS:

1. Write the names of the food groups on the bottom of the box as shown in the picture. Make sure that the grain group is on the bottom, followed by vegetables, fruits, dairy, protein and fats and sweets on the top (the same as the Food Guide Pyramid).

2. Punch six small holes along one of the long sides of the shoe box. Punch six more on the other side that pair up with the first set of holes.

3. Cut six pieces of string that are approximately twice the width of the box.

4. Knot each piece of string on one side and thread through the holes. Feed 12 beads or buttons onto each string.

5. Thread the string through the opposite hole, and tie a knot on the end to secure.

Once you have completed your **Nutrition Abacus**, use it to check your daily food habits:

■ Each time you eat a meal or snack, move a bead across for every serving that you eat from each food group. By the end of the day, you can see if the beads that you moved across resemble the shape of the pyramid. HINT: It may be easier to use the **Nutrition Abacus** once you have recorded your diet using the **Personal Pyramid** or **Pocket Tally**.

■ The **Nutrition Abacus** is also a great planning tool. Use it to check if the school menu, your after school snack or your favorite meals are "pyramid balanced."

Did you know that you may not need to eat exactly everything the pyramid tells you to? Just as we have different hair, eyes and favorite things-to-do, we also have different nutrition needs. For example, you may need more food or less food than the pyramid suggests. Some families don't eat certain foods because of their beliefs or religion. Other times, allergies or medical conditions affect the foods you can eat. Remember—the pyramid is only a guide!

WHAT'S MY SERVING SIZE?

NOTES TO EDUCATORS:

■ The activities on pages 17 and 18 will help you and the students to understand the serving size amount that the Food Guide Pyramid is referring to. It *doesn't mean* that everyone has to eat this exact amount. But it is critical to understand the concept of how much a serving is if you are trying to accurately track your diet.

■ Most children need to eat at least the minimum number of servings for proper nutrition. But many kids will need more, especially those who are active in sports and play. The best way to know how much to eat is to listen to your body! Eat until your body feels full . . . but not too full. You should feel satisfied but not overly stuffed. Discuss with children the importance of "listening" to their body to tell them how much to eat. Ask the children how it feels to eat too much, not enough, and just the right amount.

■ The serving size activities are best set up as "measuring centers." Hands-on experience measuring foods will give children a better grasp of what a "serving" really means.

■ Since everyone is touching the foods, caution the children that this is NOT an eating activity. You may want to plan this activity in conjunction with a snack or conduct it right after lunch.

■ For more ideas on measuring centers for additional foods, please refer to page 45 in the book *How to Teach Nutrition to Kids*.

SUPPLIES NEEDED:

Measuring cups
Serving utensils
Plates and bowls
Cooked pasta (soak in water beforehand to avoid sticking)
Box of ready-to-eat cereal

SERVING GUIDELINES

WHAT COUNTS AS ONE SERVING?

Breads, Cereals, Rice and Pasta
1 slice of bread
1/2 cup of cooked rice or pasta
1/2 cup of cooked cereal
1 cup of ready-to-eat cereal

Vegetables
1/2 cup of chopped raw or cooked
   vegetables
1 cup of leafy raw vegetables

Fruits
1 piece of fruit or melon wedge
3/4 cup of juice
1/2 cup of canned fruit
1/4 cup of dried fruit

Milk, Yogurt and Cheese
1 cup of milk or yogurt
1-1/2 to 2 ounces of cheese

Meat, Poultry, Fish, Dry Beans, Eggs and Nuts
2-1/2 to 3 ounces of cooked lean meat,
   poultry or fish
Count 1/2 cup of cooked beans, or 1 egg,
   or 2 tablespoons of peanut butter as 1
   ounce of lean meat (about 1/3 serving)

Fats, Oils and Sweets
LIMIT CALORIES FROM THESE
especially if you need to lose weight

NOTE: The amount you eat may be more than one serving. For example, a dinner portion of spaghetti would count as two or three servings of pasta.

Source: USDA/USDHHS

HOW MANY SERVINGS DO YOU NEED EACH DAY?

	Women & some older adults	Children, teen girls active women, most men	Teen boys & active men
Calorie level*	about 1,600	about 2,200	about 2,800
Bread group	6	9	11
Vegetable group	3	4	5
Fruit group	2	3	4
Milk group	**2–3	**2–3	**2–3
Meat group	2, for a total of 5 ounces	2, for a total of 6 ounces	3, for a total of 7 ounces

These are the calorie levels if you choose lowfat, lean foods from the 5 major food groups and use foods from the fats, oils and sweets group sparingly.

**Women who are pregnant or breastfeeding, teenagers, and young adults to age 24 need 3 servings.*

Source: USDA/USDHHS

WHAT'S YOUR SERVING SIZE OF CEREAL?

Name _____

DIRECTIONS:

1. Pretend it is breakfast time and you are hungry for your favorite cereal.

2. Using a cereal bowl, pour in the amount that you normally would eat for breakfast.

3. Using a 1/2 cup measuring cup, measure how many scoops of cereal that you just poured into your bowl. Tally it here: _____

4. Look at the product label or the chart below. What is the serving size for dry ready-to-eat cereal?

5. How many servings did you pour into your bowl?

WHAT COUNTS AS ONE SERVING?

Breads, Cereals, Rice and Pasta
1 slice of bread
1/2 cup of cooked rice or pasta
1/2 cup of cooked cereal
1 cup of ready-to-eat cereal

Vegetables
1/2 cup of chopped raw or cooked
  vegetables
1 cup of leafy raw vegetables

Fruits
1 piece of fruit or melon wedge
3/4 cup of juice
1/2 cup of canned fruit
1/4 cup of dried fruit

Milk, Yogurt and Cheese
1 cup of milk or yogurt
1-1/2 to 2 ounces of cheese

Meat, Poultry, Fish, Dry Beans, Eggs and Nuts
2-1/2 to 3 ounces of cooked lean meat,
  poultry or fish
Count 1/2 cup of cooked beans, or 1 egg,
  or 2 tablespoons of peanut butter as 1
  ounce of lean meat (about 1/3 serving)

Fats, Oils and Sweets
LIMIT CALORIES FROM THESE
especially if you need to lose weight

NOTE: The amount you eat may be more than one serving. For example, a dinner portion of spaghetti would count as two or three servings of pasta.   Source: USDA/USDHHS

It's perfectly fine to eat several servings of a food group at one meal. Remember—the Food Guide Pyramid encourages us to eat 6–11 daily servings from the grain group. The reason for this activity is to give you a better idea of how to keep track of your servings each day.

WHAT'S YOUR SERVING SIZE OF SPAGHETTI?

Name _____

DIRECTIONS:

1. Pretend it is dinner time and your family is serving spaghetti.

2. Using a dinner plate, scoop up the amount of spaghetti that you normally would eat for dinner.

3. Using a 1/2 cup measuring cup, measure how many scoops of spaghetti that you just placed on your plate. Tally it here: _____

4. Look at the chart below. What is the serving size for spaghetti (pasta)?

5. How many servings did you place on your plate?

WHAT COUNTS AS ONE SERVING?

Breads, Cereals, Rice and Pasta
1 slice of bread
1/2 cup of cooked rice or pasta
1/2 cup of cooked cereal
1 cup of ready-to-eat cereal

Vegetables
1/2 cup of chopped raw or cooked
    vegetables
1 cup of leafy raw vegetables

Fruits
1 piece of fruit or melon wedge
3/4 cup of juice
1/2 cup of canned fruit
1/4 cup of dried fruit

Milk, Yogurt and Cheese
1 cup of milk or yogurt
1-1/2 to 2 ounces of cheese

Meat, Poultry, Fish, Dry Beans, Eggs and Nuts
2-1/2 to 3 ounces of cooked lean meat,
    poultry or fish
Count 1/2 cup of cooked beans, or 1 egg,
    or 2 tablespoons of peanut butter as 1
    ounce of lean meat (about 1/3 serving)

Fats, Oils and Sweets
LIMIT CALORIES FROM THESE
especially if you need to lose weight

NOTE: The amount you eat may be more than one serving. For example, a dinner portion of spaghetti would count as two or three servings of pasta.   Source: USDA/USDHHS

It's perfectly fine to eat several servings of a food group at one meal. Remember—the Food Guide Pyramid encourages us to eat 6–11 daily servings from the grain group. The reason for this activity is to give you a better idea of how to keep track of your servings each day.

WEEKLY ACTIVITY CHECK-OFF

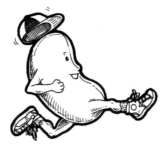

I

Name _____

Are you an active, busy kid full of energy? Or, do you sit too much in front of the television or computer?

   Every day, we have to sit still some of the time (like in school) and our bodies need daily rest (like at night).

   Other times, our bodies need to MOVE. Moving our bodies works our muscles, strengthens our heart and keeps us healthy. It can also be a whole lot of FUN!

   The chart below shows the types of activities that will keep your body cruising along at its very best. Keep track of your activities this week.

AEROBIC* ACTIVITIES:

Try for at least *3–5* each week

☐ Biking ___ minutes	☐ Hiking ___ minutes	☐ Dancing ___ minutes
☐ Running ___ minutes	☐ Cross-Country Skiing ___ minutes	☐ Jump Roping ___ minutes
☐ Swimming ___ minutes	☐ In-line Skating ___ minutes	☐ Fast Walking ___ minutes

Other aerobic activities:

_____ minutes: _____

_____ minutes: _____

_____ minutes: _____   **TOTAL AEROBIC ACTIVITIES** _____

*Aerobic activities are those which you can do at a steady pace for at least **15 minutes**. You should be breathing a little hard but you *should not* feel out of breath.

GAMES AND SPORTS:

Try for at least *1–2* each week

☐ Tag	☐ Basketball	☐ Soccer
☐ Volleyball	☐ Wall Ball	☐ Football
☐ Ice Skating	☐ Gymnastics	☐ Karate or Tae Kwondo
☐ _____	☐ _____	☐ _____
☐ _____	☐ _____	☐ _____

TOTAL GAMES AND SPORTS _____

OTHER WORK & PLAY ACTIVITIES:

Try for at least *1–2* each week

☐ Chores	☐ Gardening	☐ Bowling
☐ Golf	☐ Hopscotch	☐ Stretching
☐ Tether Ball	☐ _____	☐ _____

TOTAL WORK & PLAY _____

MY BODY IS A GREAT BODY!

Name _____

Did you know that *every* body is a great body? Bodies come in a wide variety of colors, shapes and sizes. Some of us are taller, shorter, rounder or thinner. The one thing we do all have in common is the choice to take the best care of our very own, very great body!

Answer the questions below about your great body:

The thing I like best about my body is _____

_____

My body is good at _____

_____

When my body feels rested and energetic, I like to _____

_____

When my body feels quiet and less energetic, I like to _____

_____

Some of the ways I take care of my body:

1. _____

    _____

2. _____

    _____

3. _____

    _____

4. _____

    _____

5. _____

    _____

A Picture of My Great Body:

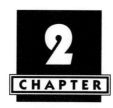

Setting Goals and Making Choices

NOTES TO EDUCATORS

Our job as nutrition educators and parents is to provide kids with the opportunity and knowledge to make healthful choices. Sometimes though, in spite of our best efforts, we observe children who make mostly poor food choices. Frustrated, we may blame ourselves for failing to properly educate children about nutrition.

But while we can offer nutrition experiences that reinforce good eating habits, provide mostly healthful food choices, and model good eating practices, the decision to put nutrition knowledge into practice ultimately lies with each *individual child*.

In this chapter, you will find activities that empower children by allowing them to set and monitor goals, make their own plans for breakfast and snack time, and role play the choices they would make in a variety of situations. In other words, the activities presented here reinforce the control that children have over their own health and nutrition.

GOAL SETTING FOR THE PRIMARY LEVEL

For younger children, the worksheet on page 26 is an introduction to goal setting. Explain to children that a goal is like a plan. Just as plans are sometimes changed or interrupted, goals may need to be modified in order to achieve success.

Setting goals is something children can apply to many areas of their life, including academics, behavior, physical fitness, nutrition and other areas of health. Parents and teachers can serve as role models by setting good health goals along with the children.

SETTING S.N.A.C.K. GOALS

Intermediate students can begin to set more specific goals that can be quantified and measured. The S.N.A.C.K. system allows the child to set effective goals that are more likely to prove successful. Encourage students to evaluate their goals to make sure they meet the criteria of S.N.A.C.K. listed on page 22.

S.N.A.C.K. GOALS

S = **Small**

Is this goal small enough so that I can meet it in a short period of time?

N = **Needed**

Is this a change that I need to make for better health?

A = **Achievable**

Can I achieve this goal? Will I need the help of others to meet this goal? Is it a goal that I can really accomplish?

C = **Can I Count it?**

Is this goal written in a way that I can count and measure my progress?

K = **Know-How**

Do I know enough to set this health goal? Where would I find more information on this topic?

GOAL SETTING

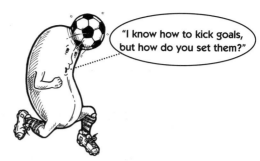

Have you sized up your diet yet using the *Personal Pyramid*, *Pocket Tally*, or *Nutrition Abacus*? Have you completed the *Weekly Activity Check-Off*? If so, you may have noticed a few changes you could make to improve your health habits.

Whenever you want to make a change, the first thing you need to do is to set a goal. The best kind of goals are ones that you can meet! If you set goals that are too hard, you may end up giving up on making changes. One way to set goals that you can meet is to use the S.N.A.C.K system:

S = Small

Is this goal small enough so that I can meet it in a short period of time?

N = Needed

Is this a change that I need to make for better health?

A = Achievable

Can I achieve this goal? Will I need the help of others to meet this goal? Is it a goal that I can really accomplish?

C = Can I Count it?

Is this goal written in a way that I can count and measure my progress?

K = Know-How

Do I know enough to set this health goal? Where would I find more information on this topic?

A great way to check your progress in meeting goals is to use the goal-setting calendar on page 24.

Q. Can you think of other ways to check your progress at meeting goals? (Some ideas are listed at the bottom of the page.)

_____

_____

_____

_____

_____

_____

A. Some ideas: bar, line or pie graphs; write a description of how you met your goal; draw a picture of how you met your goal

GOAL-SETTING CALENDAR

I

Name _____

	SUN	MON	TUE	WED	THU	FRI	SAT	MY PROGRESS:
Week 1 Dates _____ My Goal This Week: _____ _____								☐ I Met My Goal! ☐ I Still Need to Work on This: _____ _____
Week 2 Dates _____ My Goal This Week: _____ _____								☐ I Met My Goal! ☐ I Still Need to Work on This: _____ _____
Week 3 Dates _____ My Goal This Week: _____ _____								☐ I Met My Goal! ☐ I Still Need to Work on This: _____ _____
Week 4 Dates _____ My Goal This Week: _____ _____								☐ I Met My Goal! ☐ I Still Need to Work on This: _____ _____

REMEMBER TO SET S.N.A.C.K. GOALS:
SMALL, **N**EEDED, **A**CHIEVABLE, **C**AN I **C**OUNT IT?, **K**NOW-HOW

24

SAMPLE GOAL-SETTING CALENDAR

Name: **Hugh**

	SUN	MON	TUE	WED	THU	FRI	SAT	MY PROGRESS:
Week 1 Dates 4/5–4/11 My Goal This Week: **Try at least two** **new vegetables**	☒ Tried jicama— YUM!		☒ Mom put pea pods in the stir-fry			☒ At school, we had baby corn on our salad. It was OK.		☒ I Met My Goal! ☐ I Still Need to Work on This:
Week 2 Dates 4/12–4/18 My Goal This Week: **Ride my bike to my** friends houses at least twice		☒ Rode bike to Susan's	☒ Rode bike to Matt's (big hill!)			☒ Rode bike to Matt's again!		☒ I Met My Goal! ☐ I Still Need to Work on This:
Week 3 Dates 4/19–4/25 My Goal This Week: **Eat breakfast every day** this week (even if I have early band practice)	☒	☒ Band practice— I got up earlier	☒	☒ Slept in, but ate breakfast at school	☒	☒ Band practice— breakfast at school	☒	☒ I Met My Goal! ☐ I Still Need to Work on This:
Week 4 Dates 4/26–5/2 My Goal This Week: **Cut down on soda pop—** I will only drink 3 cans instead of 7	1 can at Grandma's	☒ NO SODA!	1 can	1 can at Roger's house	☒ NO SODA!	1 can (movies)	1 can	☐ I Met My Goal! ☒ I Still Need to Work on This: *I need to remember to drink water instead*

REMEMBER TO SET S.N.A.C.K. GOALS:
SMALL, **N**EEDED, **A**CHIEVABLE, **C**AN I **C**OUNT IT?, **K**NOW-HOW

MY GOALS FOR GOOD HEALTH

Name _____

This week, I will work on one of the following goals for better health:

☐ Try a new vegetable or fruit.

☐ Play active games or ride my bike after school.

☐ Eat breakfast.

☐ Choose nutritious after-school snacks.

☐ Drink water instead of sweetened drinks more often.

☐ Drink or eat three servings of foods from the **Milk**, **Yogurt**, and **Cheese** group each day.

☐ My idea for a goal: _____

_____

Draw a picture or write a story about you and your goal for good health.

"Watch me make a goal!"

BRAVO FOR BREAKFAST!

▣ Take time to wake up your brain!

Name _____

Did you know that kids who eat breakfast do better in school? That's because breakfast feeds both your body and your mind. If you are too busy to eat a healthy breakfast, try one of the following ideas:

☐ Get up 15 minutes earlier.

☐ Eat breakfast at school.

☐ Pack your breakfast in a bag and eat it on the bus.

☐ Your ideas: _____

_____

_____

My favorite breakfast is dinner! It's true! You can eat sandwiches, soup, pasta or even pizza in the morning.

Can you plan three easy, nutritious breakfasts that you can fix by yourself? Try for at least **three** different food groups in each breakfast plan:

1. _____

_____

_____

2. _____

_____

_____

3. _____

_____

_____

MAKE A SNACK PLAN

Name _____

Snacks are an important way to keep your body fueled all day long. Think of snacks as "mini-meals," made up of the same kinds of nutritious food that you eat at Breakfast, Lunch and Dinner. Below are some examples of healthy, easy-to-fix snacks:

Pretzels and string cheese

Peanut butter & fruit sandwich on whole wheat bread (try applesauce, sliced banana, or raisins)

Flavored low-fat yogurt and an orange

Wheat flakes cereal with 1% or skim milk

Now, it's your turn! In the spaces below plan three easy and nutritious snacks that you can fix by yourself. Each snack should contain at least **two** different food groups and include foods that you like!

1. _____

_____

_____

2. _____

_____

_____

3. _____

_____

_____

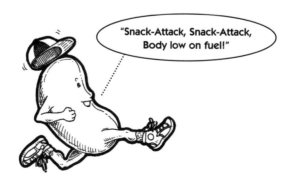

"Snack-Attack, Snack-Attack, Body low on fuel!"

A ROLE-PLAYING GAME

E Thinking Through Our Choices

NOTES TO EDUCATORS:

Role playing in small familiar groups is a great way for children to learn to think critically and solve nutrition-related problems. The following realistic scenarios allow children to practice making choices and explore the consequences of those choices. Stress that there are no right or wrong answers in these situations.

DIRECTIONS:

Copy this page and cut out the scenarios. Divide children into small groups of 2–3 and give each group a different slip. Encourage children to discuss the situation and develop brief skits that demonstrate the problem and the students' solution.

Your friend thinks she is too fat so she decides to go on a diet that she found in one of her mom's magazines. She wants you to go on the diet, too. How would you handle this situation?	You always have to rush to make it to afternoon soccer practice on time. You usually grab a can of pop and package of potato chips to eat on the way. The problem is, your stomach often starts hurting in the middle of practice, especially if you have to run a lot. What do you think is causing your stomach aches? What changes could you make to solve this problem?
After school, you always feel so hungry. When your mom's not looking, you grab a bunch of cookies and go outside to play. Later, you don't feel hungry for supper. What would you do next time you're hungry after school?	Your best friend is a picky eater who rarely eats from the five food groups. You have noticed that he looks pale and tired and gets sick a lot. What could you do to help your friend?
You like it when your Dad packs fruit, vegetable sticks, and other healthy foods in your lunch. But the kids at school tease you about eating healthy foods, calling you "vegetable head." How would you solve this problem?	Your mom is a health food nut. She is forever bringing home strange looking vegetables with even stranger-sounding names, things like bok choy, kohlrabi, and rutabaga! Worse yet, she expects you to eat them. You refuse, saying you will not try anything that looks or sounds strange. Is there a better way to deal with this situation?
Your friend says that a "Giggles" candy bar is healthy because the commercial on TV showed kids with lots of energy after they ate "Giggles." He is now convinced that "Giggles" will give him energy, too. What would you tell him?	Your big sister is pretty and popular but all she ever eats are salads and diet soft drinks. She says most other foods are "fattening." Is she right? What would you say to her?
On school mornings, you would rather sleep longer and skip breakfast. You really aren't that hungry when you first wake up, anyway. But lately, you have noticed that after morning recess, you have a headache, your stomach growls, and it's hard to do your work. How would you solve this problem?	Your parents went out for the evening, leaving you with a teenage babysitter. The babysitter says you can have whatever you want for dinner, even candy! What foods would you choose?

CHAPTER

Finding Out More About the Food You Eat

NOTES TO EDUCATORS

The activities presented in this chapter are primarily targeted to the intermediate level student. While younger students should be encouraged to begin reading food labels, students in grades three through six can begin to take a critical look at food labeling and advertising.

Sometimes we form opinions about food without knowing all the facts. One of the best ways to get a better understanding of the food we eat is to take a close look at the **Nutrition Facts** food label. The exercises on pages 32 and 33 require students to evaluate foods based on the label information and arrive at some logical conclusions. This activity works well in an individual or group setting.

Additional Nutrition Facts label information and activity ideas are presented on pages 63–69 in the book *How to Teach Nutrition to Kids*.

The "Be an Ad Buster" activities help children to take a closer look at food advertising, misleading claims, and begin to understand how to determine whether the product lives up to the information in the ad.

For a more thorough background on food advertising, please see pages 110–116 in *How to Teach Nutrition to Kids*.

As children and their families rely more on fast food restaurants, it is important for children to begin to understand the nutrient content of fast food menu items and to learn to make more healthful choices, at least some of the time.

Most fast food restaurants have nutrient information available that you can request. Make available several nutrition information brochures from popular restaurants. Before students begin this activity, review the general guidelines for fast food meal planning included on the "Not So Fast..." worksheet on page 36 (600–800 calories, 20–27 grams of fat, and at least three food groups represented). This activity works well in individual or group settings.

LABEL LOGIC

 Potatoes

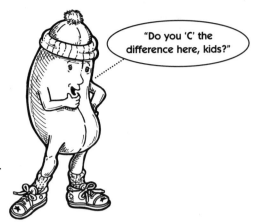

"Do you 'C' the difference here, kids?"

Name _____

FAT AND VITAMIN C

Potatoes are a very healthy vegetable. They are high in carbohydrate, fiber and vitamin C. Not all foods made from potatoes are equal in nutrition, though. This activity will help you to see how processing affects the nutrition of potatoes.

DIRECTIONS:

Use the Nutrition Facts food labels to complete the information about each type of potato product. Use this information to answer the questions that follow.

Fried Potato Crisps			**Baked Potato**			**Hashed Brown Potatoes**			**French Fries**			**Mashed Potatoes**		
Serving Size 1 oz. (28g)			Serving Size 1 medium (with skin)			Serving Size 1/2 cup (78g)			Serving Size 10 (50g)			Serving Size 1/2 cup (105g)		
Amount Per Serving			**Amount Per Serving**			**Amount Per Serving**			**Amount Per Serving**			**Amount Per Serving**		
Calories 158	Calories from Fat 99		**Calories** 150	Calories from Fat 0		**Calories** 163	Calories from Fat 99		**Calories** 158	Calories from Fat 72		**Calories** 111	Calories from Fat 36	
		% Daily Value*			% Daily Value*			% Daily Value*			% Daily Value*			% Daily Value*
Total Fat 11g		17%	**Total Fat** 0g		0%	**Total Fat** 11g		17%	**Total Fat** 8g		12%	**Total Fat** 4g		6%
Saturated Fat 3g		15%	**Saturated Fat** 0g		0%	**Saturated Fat** 4g		20%	**Saturated Fat** 3g		15%	**Saturated Fat** 1g		5%
Cholesterol 0 mg		0%	**Cholesterol** 0 mg		0%	**Cholesterol** 0 mg		0%	**Cholesterol** 0 mg		0%	**Cholesterol** 13 mg		4%
Sodium 186 mg		8%	**Sodium** 11 mg		<1%	**Sodium** 19 mg		1%	**Sodium** 108 mg		5%	**Sodium** 309 mg		13%
Total Carbohydrate 14g		5%	**Total Carbohydrate** 35g		12%	**Total Carbohydrate** 17g		6%	**Total Carbohydrate** 20g		7%	**Total Carbohydrate** 18g		6%
Dietary Fiber 1g		4%	**Dietary Fiber** 3g		12%	**Dietary Fiber** 0g		0%	**Dietary Fiber** 2g		8%	**Dietary Fiber** 1g		4%
Sugars			**Sugars** 2g			**Sugars**			**Sugars**			**Sugars** 4g		
Protein 2g		4%	**Protein** 3g		6%	**Protein** 2g		4%	**Protein** 2g		4%	**Protein** 2g		4%
Vitamin A		<2%	Vitamin A		<2%	Vitamin A		<2%	Vitamin A		<2%	Vitamin A		4%
Vitamin C		4%	Vitamin C		30%	Vitamin C		8%	Vitamin C		8%	Vitamin C		10%
Calcium		<2%	Calcium		<2%	Calcium		<2%	Calcium		<2%	Calcium		3%
Iron		2%	Iron		10%	Iron		4%	Iron		2%	Iron		2%
*Percent Daily Values are based on a 2,000 calorie diet.			*Percent Daily Values are based on a 2,000 calorie diet.			*Percent Daily Values are based on a 2,000 calorie diet.			*Percent Daily Values are based on a 2,000 calorie diet.			*Percent Daily Values are based on a 2,000 calorie diet.		

Grams of fat/
one serving _____

Vitamin C _____
(% Daily Value)

Grams of fat/
one serving _____

Vitamin C _____
(% Daily Value)

Grams of fat/
one serving _____

Vitamin C _____
(% Daily Value)

Grams of fat/
one serving _____

Vitamin C _____
(% Daily Value)

Grams of fat/
one serving _____

Vitamin C _____
(% Daily Value)

1. Compare the fat content of the different types of potato products. Rank them from lowest to highest.

2. Compare the vitamin C content of the different types of potato products. Rank them from lowest to highest.

3. What happens to the vitamin C in a potato when it is processed into other products?

4. Which of the potato products do you think is the most nutritious? Explain how you came up with this answer.

Ready-to-Eat Cereals

Name _____

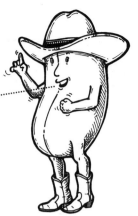

"Fiber is good stuff! It works like a broom to sweep out your digestive system."

SUGAR AND FIBER

The purpose of this exercise is to see what happens to the fiber content of breakfast cereal as the sugar content increases.

YOU WILL NEED:

A sweetened and unsweetened variety of the same type of cereal, such as Wheaties and Frosted Wheaties, Cheerios and Honey-Nut Cheerios, or Shredded Wheat and Frosted Mini-Wheats

DIRECTIONS:

Find the **Nutrition Facts** label panel on each box of cereal. Use the information to answer the questions that follow.

1. Which cereal has the most sugar in one serving? Which has the least?

_____

_____

2. Which cereal has the most fiber in one serving? Which has the least?

_____

_____

3. When extra sugar is added to a cereal, does the amount of fiber seem to increase or decrease? Why?

_____

_____

4. Do you think it is a good idea to add sugar to breakfast cereal? Why or why not?

_____

_____

ACTIVITY IDEA

YOU WILL NEED:

Table sugar, 1/4 teaspoon measuring spoon, colored plates, a variety of ready-to-eat cereal boxes

DIRECTIONS:

One-fourth teaspoon of sugar is equal to one gram of sugar. For each type of cereal, look at the label and find out how many grams of sugar are in one serving. Use the 1/4 teaspoon to measure the grams of sugar in each type of cereal. Display on a colored plate beside the box. Does the amount of sugar in some cereals surprise you?

BE AN AD-BUSTER

I Analyzing "Frooty-Tooty Fruitsies"

Name _____

Did you know that food advertising can sometimes make a food sound more nutritious than it really is? You need to take a close look at the food label to determine if the food lives up to the advertising claims.

DIRECTIONS:

Read the advertisement for "Frooty-Tooty Fruitsies." (It's made-up, by the way.) Next, study the **Nutrition Facts** label for this product and answer the questions below.

WHAT THE ADVERTISEMENT SAYS:

Frooty-Tooty Fruitsies give your body a high-energy boost. They are bursting with FRUIT flavor and wholesome goodness. Frooty-Tooty Fruitsies make a Fruity-Licious Nutritious Treat!!

WHAT THE LABEL SHOWS:

Frooty-Tooty Fruitsies

Serving Size 15 pieces
Servings Per Container 1

Amount Per Serving

Calories 120   Calories from Fat 0

	% Daily Value*
Total Fat 0g	0%
Saturated Fat 0g	0%
Cholesterol 0 mg	0%
Sodium 45 mg	2%
Total Carbohydrate 29g	10%
Dietary Fiber 0g	0%
Sugars 23g	
Protein 1g	2%
Vitamin A	<2%
Vitamin C	<2%
Calcium	<2%
Iron	<2%

*Percent Daily Values are based on a 2,000 calorie diet.

Ingredients:
Corn syrup, sugar, gelatin, fruit juice concentrate, artificial flavorings, artificial colorings.

---

1. The ingredients on a food label are listed from most to least. Look at the ingredient label for **Frooty-Tooty Fruitsies**. How many of the first three ingredients are forms of sugar? Are any of the ingredients listed a source of real fruit?

   _____

2. Real fruit and 100% fruit juices often contribute vitamins A and C to the diet. Are **Frooty-Tooty Fruitsies** a good source of either of these vitamins?

   _____

3. Do you think that **Frooty-Tooty Fruitsies** are a "Fruity-licious Nutritious" treat? Why or why not?

   _____

   _____

4. Can you think of an example of a food advertisement that you have seen that makes misleading claims about nutrition? Describe below.

   _____

   _____

BE AN AD-BUSTER

I̲ A Closer Look at Saturday Morning TV

Name _____

DIRECTIONS:

To complete this activity, you will watch at least one hour of Saturday morning programming on a commercial television network, such as ABC, CBS, NBC, Fox or Nickelodeon. Once you decide on the channel, do not switch networks until you have finished this assignment.

Network Watched _____   What Time Did You Start Watching? _____

Date Watched _____   What Time Did You Stop Watching? _____

Every time you see a food commercial, make a tally mark beside the category below that best describes the food advertised.

_____ Candy

_____ Pop

_____ Sweetened beverages
                (not 100% fruit juice)

_____ Sweetened cereal

_____ Corn chips, potato chips, or other
                fried snacks

_____ Cakes, cookies, or pastries

_____ Sweetened fruit snacks

_____ Other sweetened foods

FOOD GROUPS:

_____ Grain (breads, low-sugar cereals, waffles, pasta, rice)

_____ Fruit (fresh, frozen, or canned, 100% fruit juices)

_____ Vegetables (fresh, frozen, or canned, vegetable juices)

_____ Protein (meat, fish, chicken, beans, eggs, peanut butter)

_____ Dairy (milk, cheese, yogurt)

OTHERS:

_____ Combination Meals (examples: pizza, children's frozen dinners)

_____ Fast food restaurants

_____ Public Service Announcements promoting good nutrition

_____ _____

_____ _____

How many total food advertisements did you see during the time you watched? _____

How many of these were for foods that you consider nutritious? _____

How many of these were for foods that are not the most nutritious? _____

Do you think there should be more advertisements for healthy foods on television?

Why or why not? _____

_____

NOT SO FAST... MAKE A GAME PLAN FOR EATING OUT

Name _____

Planning ahead is the key to eating more nutritious meals at fast food restaurants. The nutrition advice in the box below will help you to plan a more balanced meal. For each menu that you plan, try to stay within the calorie, fat, and food group guidelines.

Menu Planning Guidelines
☐ 600–800 total calories for one meal
☐ 20–27 grams of fat for one meal
☐ At least three food groups represented in each meal

DID YOU KNOW?

■ Many restaurants publish the nutrition information for the food items they serve. To get a copy, all you need to do is ask!

■ If you choose a meal that is high in fat or calories, be sure to balance your food choices during the rest of the day.

EXAMPLE

RESTAURANT: Taco Bell

Food Item	Calories	Fat grams	Food groups
Chicken Burrito	345	13	Meat, Grain, Dairy
Salsa	27	0	Vegetable
Seasoned Rice	110	3	Grain
Cinnamon Crisps	139	6	Grain, (Fats/Sweets)
TOTALS:	621	22	4 different groups

See next page for sample sheets to copy and fill out.

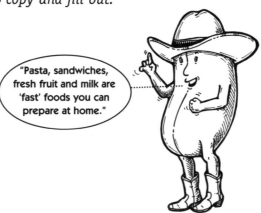

"Pasta, sandwiches, fresh fruit and milk are 'fast' foods you can prepare at home."

RESTAURANT: _____

Food Item	Calories	Fat grams	Food groups

TOTALS:

- -

RESTAURANT: _____

Food Item	Calories	Fat grams	Food groups

TOTALS:

- -

RESTAURANT: _____

Food Item	Calories	Fat grams	Food groups

TOTALS:

CHAPTER

Cooking Up Some Fun

NOTES TO EDUCATORS

Cooking projects are one of the most memorable and relevant methods to teach children about food and nutrition. The recipes on the following pages allow children to creatively experiment within a basic framework of tried-and-true recipes. Most of the recipes in this chapter can be prepared by kids of all ages. Younger children will need closer supervision, however.

Whether cooking at home or at school, it is always important to stress the importance of being safe and sanitary when handling food. **Always** instruct children to wash their hands before cooking and whenever they use the restroom or touch their hair, nose, or neighbor. Closely supervise the children's use of knives, equipment, microwaves, ovens, and other cooking surfaces. The appendix on pages 160–162 in *How to Teach Nutrition to Kids* offers specific guidance for keeping cooking projects safe and sanitary.

Creative cooking projects also make great homework assignments. Encourage students to try one of the recipes suggested here or create one of their own. The *Recipe Evaluation Form* on page 46 should be completed for each recipe that you assign.

NOTE: Look for other recipes on the bottom of the food group puzzle sheets in Chapter 5.

WACKY SNACK 1

 Tortilla + Pizza = TORTIZZA!

"A Wacky-Snack is when you mix two or more foods together and get a delicious snack with a funny name."

Name _____

INGREDIENTS:

1 10" whole wheat flour tortilla

2 T. prepared pasta sauce

1/4 cup grated part-skim mozzarella cheese

1/4 cup chopped vegetables of your choice
    (e.g. red pepper, mushrooms, onions, broccoli florets, grated carrots, diced tomatoes, olives, etc.)

DIRECTIONS:

Spread sauce evenly over tortilla. Add remaining ingredients and roll into a burrito-type shape. Microwave on high for 1 minute.

Makes 1 serving

My Wacky Snack Recipe:

_____ + _____ = _____

INGREDIENTS:

_____

_____

_____

_____

DIRECTIONS:

_____

_____

_____

_____

WACKY SNACK 2

 ## Burrito + Potato = BURRATO!

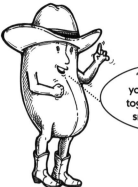

"A Wacky-Snack is when you mix two or more foods together and get a delicious snack with a funny name"

Name _____

INGREDIENTS:

1 medium potato
2 T. refried beans
1-2 T. salsa
2 T. grated reduced-fat cheddar cheese

DIRECTIONS:

Clean and scrub potato. Using a sharp knife, carefully poke the potato (this allows the steam to escape during cooking). Microwave on high for 6–7 minutes. After the potato has cooled, cut in half, press down to flatten, and spread remaining ingredients in the groove. Microwave on high for 1 minute.

Makes 1 serving

My Wacky Snack Recipe:

_____ + _____ = _____

INGREDIENTS:

_____
_____
_____
_____

DIRECTIONS:

_____
_____
_____
_____

41

WACKY SNACK 3

 Human + Banana = HUBANA!

Name _____

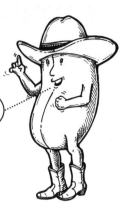

"A Wacky-Snack is when you mix two or more foods together and get a delicious snack with a funny name"

INGREDIENTS:

Banana
Peanut butter or reduced-fat cream cheese
Dried apricot half
Grated carrots (optional)
Raisins, dried cranberries, or other dried fruits of choice
Shelled sunflower seeds

DIRECTIONS:

Peel banana half-way down. On the very top, place a dab of peanut butter or cream cheese and place the apricot half on top. This is the beret or hat. If you prefer, place grated carrots on the peanut butter for hair. Dab peanut butter on the banana where you want the eyes, nose, and mouth to go. Stick on sunflower seeds, raisins, dried cranberries, or other fruit to make the face. Say "Hi" to your hubana, take a picture if you wish, and then EAT!

Makes 1 serving

My Wacky Snack Recipe:

_____ + _____ = _____

INGREDIENTS:

_____

_____

_____

_____

DIRECTIONS:

_____

_____

_____

_____

_____

42

MAKE YOUR OWN RECIPE

 Egg-Xactly Right Eggs

Name _____

This recipe is a fool-proof way for the beginning cook to learn to make fluffy scrambled eggs.

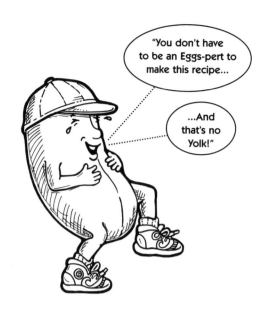

"You don't have to be an Eggs-pert to make this recipe...

...And that's no Yolk!"

Basic Recipe

INGREDIENTS:
4 medium eggs
1/4 cup nonfat or 1% milk
non-stick spray
salt & pepper to taste

EQUIPMENT:
1 mixing bowl, 1 microwave dish with lid, wire whisk or fork

DIRECTIONS:
Spray the microwave dish with non-stick spray. Crack the eggs in the mixing bowl, add milk and stir well with wire whisk or fork. Pour into microwave dish, cover and microwave on high for 4 minutes. Carefully remove eggs from the microwave using pot holders. Remove the lid and use a spoon to break the eggs into bite-sized pieces. Add a small amount of salt and pepper or try one of the variations below. Be creative!

Makes 2 servings

VARIATIONS:

Eggs Ole'—After you remove eggs from the microwave, top with 2 tablespoons of salsa, 5 sliced black olives, and 2 tablespoons of grated cheddar cheese. Replace lid and let eggs sit for 1–2 more minutes.

Greek Eggs—Add 1/2 tsp. of oregano to the basic recipe prior to cooking. After you remove eggs from the microwave, top with 2 tablespoons of fresh, chopped tomato and 2–3 tablespoons of feta cheese. Replace lid and let eggs sit for 1–2 more minutes.

Pita Pocket Veggie Breakfast—Stuff a pita pocket with scrambled eggs, 2 tablespoons of grated mozzarella or jack cheese, and chopped vegetables of your choice such as onions, green pepper, broccoli or sun-dried tomatoes.

My Own Egg-Xactly Right Egg Variations:

_____

_____

_____

_____

MAKE YOUR OWN RECIPE

I Soup Your Way!

Name _____

The possibilities are endless for creating variations of this delicious, Italian soup!

Pick **ONE** choice in each category for this recipe:

Broth* (2 cups): ☐ Vegetable   ☐ Chicken   ☐ Beef

Juice* (3 cups): ☐ Vegetable juice   ☐ Tomato juice

Vegetables: ☐ 1 pound bag of frozen peas, corn, green beans or various mixed vegetable combinations

☐ 3–4 cups fresh cut-up vegetables such as carrots, potatoes, zucchini or cabbage

☐ Combination of frozen and fresh vegetables (3–4 cups total)

Protein: ☐ 1 can (approximately 16 ounces) kidney, pinto, white or black beans, drained*

☐ 2 cups of lean meat, such as cut-up turkey or ham, or cooked ground beef

Pasta: ☐ 1 cup of your favorite shaped pasta such as macaroni, small shells, rotini or bowties

☐ 1/2 teaspoon garlic powder
☐ 1 tsp. Italian seasoning
☐ 1/2 tsp. pepper
☐ 1 cup water

*May substitute low-sodium varieties of these ingredients

DIRECTIONS:

In large saucepan, combine broth, juice, vegetables, protein ingredient, water, garlic, Italian seasoning, and pepper. Cook on medium heat until soup boils. Add pasta and cook for 15–20 minutes, until pasta is tender.

Makes 8–10 servings

HINT: To make the meal complete, just add whole-grain bread or crackers, fresh fruit and sliced or grated low-fat cheese.

Notes on My Favorite Ingredients for this recipe _____

_____

_____

_____

MAKE YOUR OWN RECIPE

E Fuel-Up Trail Mix

Name _____

Fuel-up Trail Mix makes a great snack to put in your backpack, gym bag or the car. It is delicious and easy to make!

Using a 1/4 cup measuring cup, mix equal amounts of some or all of the following ingredients (Choose the ones you like!)

- ☐ Low-fat granola cereal
- ☐ Quick-cooking oatmeal
- ☐ Low-sugar breakfast cereal
- ☐ Small Pretzel sticks or twists
- ☐ Shelled Sunflower seeds
- ☐ Peanuts
- ☐ Almonds
- ☐ Raisins
- ☐ Dried cranberries
- ☐ Dried apple rings
- ☐ Dried apricots
- ☐ Dried blueberries
- ☐ Other dried fruits:
- ☐ _____
- ☐ _____
- ☐ _____

Mix in 1-2 tablespoons of **ONE** of the following:

- ☐ Chocolate chips
- ☐ Candy coated peanuts
- ☐ Other small candies

My Very Own, Very Favorite Trail Mix Combination:

_____

_____

_____

_____

_____

_____

_____

RECIPE EVALUATION FORM

"This is homework the dog **really** could eat!"

Name _____

DIRECTIONS:

Ask your teacher for copies of the *Wacky Snacks* or *Make Your Own Recipe* sheets.
Pick a recipe that you would like to try or use a recipe idea of your own.

Always ask permission from an adult before you start! When you are finished, be sure to complete this worksheet.

GOOD COOK REMINDERS!

Every time I cook, I need to remember to:

1. Ask permission.
2. Wash my hands and work area.
3. Gather all of the ingredients.

4. Gather all of the equipment.
5. Prepare the recipe.
6. Clean up my work area.

7. Fill out this worksheet.

The Recipe I tried at home was: _____

This is how I made this recipe:

_____

_____

This is how it looked:

_____

_____

This is how it tasted:

_____

_____

Changes to try the next time I make this recipe:

_____

_____

_____ tasted my recipe.

                  Adult Signature

Adult comments are welcome: _____

_____

_____

5

CHAPTER

Puzzles, Activities & More Recipes

NOTES TO EDUCATORS

The activities in this chapter are a fun way to introduce a nutrition unit or reinforce nutrition concepts. Use as handouts in the cafeteria, at health fairs or during wellness week. The sheets also work well as homework assignments that children can share with their family. Encourage children to try the simple recipes included on the activity pages. Remind students to complete the recipe evaluation form on page 46.

IN THIS CHAPTER:

Use Your Brain to Find
   the Grains
Veggie Plant Parts
Fruit: Nature's Sweet Treats
The Protein Scene
A M-O-O-O-O-VING Story
   About Milk
A Month of Fitness & Fun!

PUZZLE SOLUTIONS

USE YOUR BRAIN TO FIND THE GRAINS

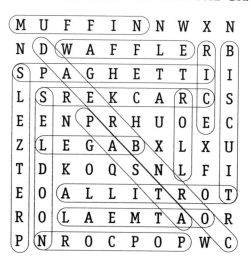

VEGGIE PLANT PARTS

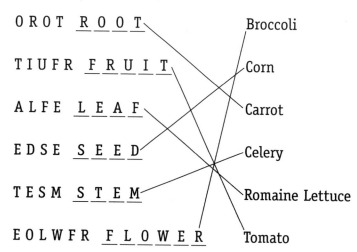

FRUIT: NATURE'S SWEET TREATS

SOME FRUITS . . .

. . . GROW ON TREES LIKE THESE:

PAPELS <u>A P P L E S</u>

ECHPAES <u>P E A C H E S</u>

SRAEP <u>P E A R S</u>

. . . GROW JUST FINE ON A VINE:

PGARES <u>G R A P E S</u>

WIKIRTIUF <u>K I W I F R U I T</u>

. . . HANG AROUND ON THE GROUND:

TWMLAREEON <u>W A T E R M E L O N</u>

ENPPPAELI <u>P I N E A P P L E</u>

RBSWARTESIER <u>S T R A W B E R R I E S</u>

. . . FEEL PUSHED TO HANG ON A BUSH:

SIRBUBLEERE <u>B L U E B E R R I E S</u>

RSBRISEREPA <u>R A S P B E R R I E S</u>

THE PROTEIN SCENE

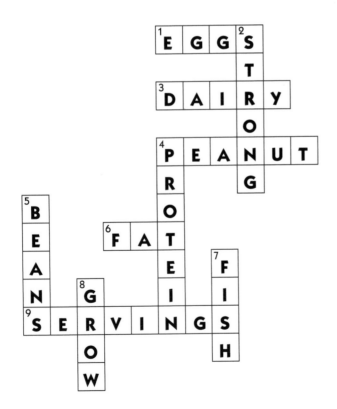

USE YOUR BRAIN TO FIND THE GRAINS!

Name _____

```
M U F F I N N W X N
N D W A F F L E R B
S P A G H E T T I I
L S R E K C A R C S
E E N P R H U O E C
Z L E G A B X L X U
T D K O Q S N L F I
E O A L L I T R O T
R O L A E M T A O R
P N R O C P O P W C
```

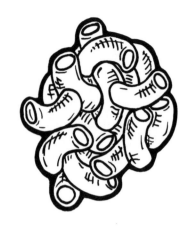

WORD LIST:

BAGEL, BISCUIT, CORNBREAD, CRACKERS, MUFFIN, NOODLES, OATMEAL, PASTA, POPCORN, PRETZELS, RICE, ROLL, SPAGHETTI, TORTILLA, WAFFLE

YUMMY EXTRA-SPECIAL OATMEAL

This oatmeal is fancy enough to serve on special occasions.

Ingredients:

2 cups water
1 c. quick-cooking oats
1 T. raisins
1 c. peeled, diced peach
   (or diced canned peaches)
1/8 tsp. ground cinnamon

1/8 tsp. ground ginger
2 T. apple juice
2 tsp. maple syrup
2 T. brown sugar
1/4 cup skim or 1% milk

Directions:

Combine first 3 ingredients in a medium sized pot and stir well. Bring to a boil over medium-high heat. Reduce heat and simmer, uncovered, for 6 minutes.

Combine peach and the next 4 ingredients in a small sized pot. Bring to a boil over medium-high heat. Reduce heat and simmer for 6 minutes.

Add brown sugar to oatmeal mixture and stir well. Divide oatmeal evenly between two serving bowls. Top each with 2 tablespoons of milk and half of the peach mixture. Serve immediately.

Makes 2 servings

VEGGIE PLANT PARTS

Name _____

Did you know that vegetables come from all parts of the plant?
Vegetables can be roots, stems, leaves, seeds, flowers or even fruit.*

DIRECTIONS:

Unscramble the part of the plant on the left column. Next,
draw a line from the plant part to the correct vegetable.

O R O T _ _ _ _ _   Broccoli

T I U F R _ _ _ _ _ _   Corn

A L F E _ _ _ _ _   Carrot

E D S E _ _ _ _ _   Celery

T E S M _ _ _ _ _   Romaine Lettuce

WORD LIST:

E O L W F R _ _ _ _ _ _ _   Tomato

Flower, Fruit, Leaf, Root, Seed, Stem

*Yes, vegetables can actually be the "fruit" part of the plant. A botanist (a scientist who studies plants) classifies
the fruit of the plant as the part that surrounds the seeds. Examples of vegetables that are the fruit part of the
plant include zucchini, cucumbers, peppers, tomatoes and eggplant.*

PLANT PART ART
A Science Project You Can Eat!

Ingredients:

Large Flat Cracker   *1 celery stick*
Peanut butter or low-fat cream cheese   *1 lettuce leaf, torn into small pieces*
2–3 broccoli florets   *1 T. grated carrots*

Directions:

Lightly spread cracker with either peanut butter or cream cheese. Next, create a plant or garden
design on the cracker by arranging shredded carrots for roots, celery stick for the stem, lettuce
for leaves and broccoli for flowers. EAT & ENJOY!

Serves 1

FRUIT: NATURE'S SWEET TREATS

Name _____

Fruit is a healthy treat that is yummy-sweet. Fruits grow many different ways and in many different places.

DIRECTIONS:
Unscramble the fruits to find out how they grow.

SOME FRUITS . . .

. . . GROW ON TREES LIKE THESE:

PAPELS __ __ __ __ __ __

ECHPAES __ __ __ __ __ __ __

SRAEP __ __ __ __ __

. . . GROW JUST FINE ON A VINE:

PGARES __ __ __ __ __ __

WIKIRTIUF __ __ __ __ __ __ __ __ __

. . . HANG AROUND ON THE GROUND:

TWMLAREEON __ __ __ __ __ __ __ __ __ __

ENPPPAELI __ __ __ __ __ __ __ __ __

RBSWARTESIER __ __ __ __ __ __ __ __ __ __ __ __

. . . FEEL PUSHED TO HANG ON A BUSH:

SIRBUBLEERE __ __ __ __ __ __ __ __ __ __ __

RSBRISEREPA __ __ __ __ __ __ __ __ __ __ __

WORD LIST:

Apples, blueberries, grapes, kiwifruit, peaches, pears, pineapple, raspberries, strawberries, watermelon

---

Family Research Idea:

What kind of plants do the following fruits grow on? **Carambola (star fruit), Guava, Papaya, Mangos, Persimmon.** Ask your parents or teacher to help you find the answers at the library or on the internet.

MAKE-YOUR-OWN FRUIT KEBABS

Ingredients:
Wooden skewers
Different kinds of cut up fruit (you choose!)

Whole berries and grapes
Nonfat vanilla yogurt

Directions:
Place fruit pieces on wooden skewers. Use your creativity to make beautiful designs and patterns! Dip in yogurt and eat. YUM!

THE PROTEIN SCENE

Name _____

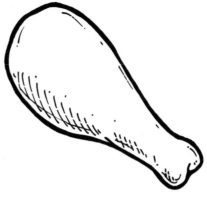

ACROSS:

1. Some kids like them scrambled.

3. Next door to the Meat/Protein Group on the Food Guide Pyramid

4. Grind this nut into butter for a popular sandwich filling.

6. Lean meats and chicken without skin are low in _____.

9. For good health, eat 2–3 _____ of protein-rich foods each day.

DOWN:

2. Foods from the Meat, Poultry, Fish, Dry Beans, Eggs & Nuts Group help to build a _____ body.

4. A nutrient that provides the building blocks for growth.

5. Hugh-Man's favorite. You can find these in burritos.

7. A protein food that lives in the water.

8. Get bigger.

WORD LIST:
Beans, Dairy, Eggs, Fat, Fish, Grow, Peanut, Protein, Servings, Strong

---

EASY LENTIL CHILI

This recipe can be served as a thick, hearty soup, as a filling for tortillas or as a topping for baked potatoes.

Ingredients:

1 pound lentils, rinsed

5 cups water

1 can tomato sauce (15 oz.)

1/2 cup chopped onion

3 teaspoons chili powder

1/2 teaspoon salt (optional)

1 cup grated cheddar cheese

Directions:

Combine lentils and water in a large pan. Place on the stove and bring to a boil. Turn the heat down, cover with a lid, and simmer for 30 minutes. Add tomato sauce, onion, chili powder and salt. Simmer for 30 minutes more. Top each serving bowl with 2 tablespoons of grated cheddar cheese.

Makes 6–8 servings

A M-O-O-O-O-VING STORY ABOUT MILK

Name _____

DIRECTIONS:

1. Answer the questions below.

2. Use the words from this page to fill in the story on
the following page.

Note: NO peeking at the story before you answer the questions!

Name a type of truck _____

A

Favorite variety of cheese _____

B

Your best friend's name _____

C

Favorite animal _____

D

Favorite sport _____

E

Name a material that is very hard _____

F

Favorite holiday _____

G

The type of milk that you usually drink _____

H

Favorite song _____

I

The month of your birthday _____

J

Town where you live _____

K

Favorite color _____

L

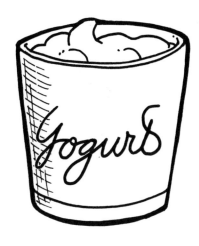

BANANA SMOOTHIE

Ingredients:

1 banana
3/4 cup lowfat milk
1/2 cup lowfat vanilla yogurt
1/4 cup orange juice

Directions:

Place ingredients in blender. Blend
until smooth and creamy. Serve
chilled.

Makes 2 cups.

53

A M-O-O-O-O-VING STORY ABOUT MILK

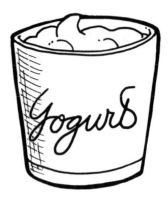

Name _____

Cruising along in my _____ on the narrow, winding roads of
                                  A

Mount _____, I suddenly came across a _____ cow.
            B   L

Right beside her was a _____, singing _____ as loudly
                            D   I

as he could. When the _____ saw me, he stopped, stared at me for a
                                D

moment, and asked me what I was carrying in my _____.
                                                    A

    I replied, "I have a load of dairy products that I'm delivering to _____,
                                                                  K

just in time for the _____ celebration. Did you know that those
                                G

folks always celebrate _____ in _____?"
                              G   J

    The cow, who introduced herself as _____, was very pleased that
                                                C

I was carrying _____ milk, yogurt and cheese in my truck. She asked
                                H

me if I knew why dairy products were important for good health.

    The _____ interrupted, anxious to tell me that dairy foods have a
                              D

lot of calcium, a nutrient that makes bones as strong as _____.
                                                      F

_____ agreed and also mentioned that you need strong bones to do
                  C

your best at _____.
                            E

    After a snack of crackers, grapes and _____, I said goodbye and
                                                      B

rushed along on my way to _____, delivering my goods just in
                                     K

time for _____.
                    G

A MONTH OF FITNESS & FUN!

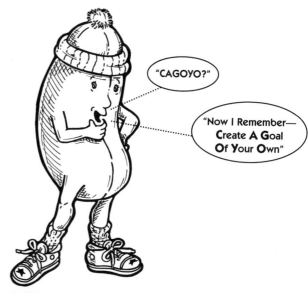

"CAGOYO?"

"Now I Remember—
Create A Goal
Of Your Own"

Name _____

Month _____

DIRECTIONS:
Mark an "X" in the square for each day that
you complete the suggested activity.

SUN	MON	TUE	WED	THU	FRI	SAT
Try a new fruit today.	Walk your dog for at least 15 min. (No dog? Borrow one!)	CAGOYO	Try a new recipe (ask an adult for permission first).	Offer to carry in groceries for an elderly person.	Make up your own active game.	Plan next week's breakfast menus.
Set up an aerobic obstacle course in your yard or play area.	Visit the Dole Web site at www.dole5aday.com	Try a new vegetable today.	Put on your chef hat and help make dinner tonight.	CAGOYO	Ask a friend to ride bikes together.	Look through gardening catalogs & pick a new vegetable to grow.
Create a commercial for a healthy food.	CAGOYO	Eat breakfast at school today.	Try a new grain today. (How about quinoa or couscous?)	Read a book about healthy eating.	Play "broom" hockey with your friends.	Get your whole family moving on a walk.
Send away for "10 Tips to Healthy Eating & Physical Activity for You"*	Play an active game after school today.	Make a fruit or vegetable pinata. Fill it with healthy prizes.	Combine yogurt & fresh fruit for a yummy after-school treat.	Visit the Kids Food Cyber Club at www.kidsfood.org	CAGOYO	Invent a new jump rope rhyme. Try it out with your friends.

*To receive a free copy of "10 Tips to Healthy Eating and Physical Activity for You," send a self-addressed stamped envelope to "10 Tips for You," P.O. Box 1144, Rockville, MD 20854.

55

APPENDIX

Hugh's Favorite Web Sites

Children's Books With Food Themes

Copy-Ready Hugh-Art

- **Hugh-Man and the Foodettes (Puppets)**

- **My Favorite Foods-to-Eat and Things-to-Do**

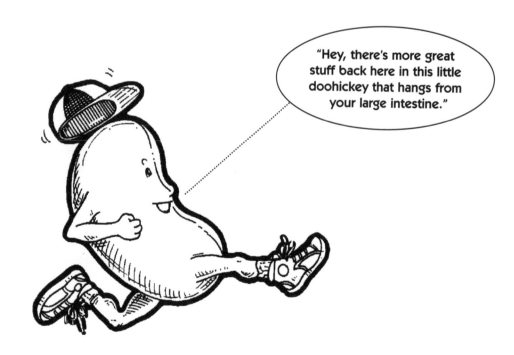

"Hey, there's more great stuff back here in this little doohickey that hangs from your large intestine."

HUGH'S FAVORITE WEB SITES

SITES FOR KIDS

Dole 5-A-Day Site
http://www.dole5aday.com

Fun Food for Kids
http://www.nppc.org/foodfun.html

Kid Food Cyber Club
http://www.kidsfood.org

Kidshealth.org
http://www.kidshealth.org/kid/food/index.html

Nutrition Cafe Game
http://www.exhibits.pacsci.org/nutrition

PearBear Healthy Kids
http://www.usapears.com/pears/pbbear.htm

Take Aim game
http://www.eatsmart.org/html/game.html

ESPECIALLY FOR TEACHERS
Nutrition Expedition
http://www.fsci.umn.edu/nutrexp

Schoolhouse: Health: Nutrition Education
http://teacherpathfinder.org/School/Subjects/Health/nutried.html

Teachnet
http://www.teachnet.com

SOMETHING FOR EVERYONE
Food & Nutrition Newsletter
http://www.ext.vt.edu/news/periodicals/foods

Food for Health Newsletter
http://www.foodforhealth.com

Iowa State Extension
http://www.exnet.iastate.edu/Pages/families/fs/homepage.htm

Jean Fremont's Food & Nutrition Page
http://www.sfu.ca/~jfremont

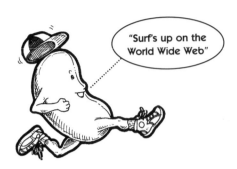

"Surf's up on the World Wide Web"

Nutrition for Kids (Hosted by *24 Carrot Press*!)
http://www.nutritionforkids.com

University of Nebraska-Lincoln Nutrition Education Site
http://www.ianr.unl.edu/nep

USDA Food & Nutrition Information Center
http://www.nal.usda.gov/fnic

USDA School Meals Initiative for Healthy School Meals
http://schoolmeals.nalusda.gov:8001

Washington State Dairy Council
http://www.eatsmart.org

PROFESSIONAL RESOURCES
American Dietetic Association
http://www.eatright.org

American School Food Service Association
http://www.asfsa.org

Arizona Health Sciences Library Nutrition Guide
http://www.ahsc.arizona.edu/nutrition

Dietetics Online
http://www.dietetics.com

National Food Service Management Institute
http://www.olemiss.edu/depts/nfsmi

CHILDREN'S BOOKS WITH FOOD THEMES

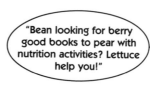

"Bean looking for berry good books to pear with nutrition activities? Lettuce help you!"

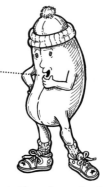

EARLY CHILDHOOD (PRESCHOOL–2ND GRADE)

Bread is For Eating

by David and Phillis Gershator, Illustrated by
Emma Shaw-Smith, Henry Holt and Company, Inc., 1995, ISBN 0-8050-3173-1

Spiritual and heart-warming, this book beautifully captures the nourishment that bread gives us. All phases of bread production are simply and elegantly presented with colorful characters and illustrations. The phrase "El pan es para comer" (translation: Bread is so good to eat) is repeated throughout with the complete song included at the end.

Grandpa's Garden Lunch

by Judith Caseley, Greenwillow Books, 1990, ISBN 0-688-08816-3

This is a delightful story of how Sarah and her Grandpa spend time together planning their garden, visiting the nursery to select plants and seeds, planting and caring for their garden and finally, eating their garden. It warmly illustrates the connection between growing a garden and eating the results!

Mealtime (Early Preschool–K)

by Maureen Roffey, Macmillan Publishing Company, 1989, ISBN 0-02-777151-2

This picture book is appropriate for even the youngest preschooler. Hand washing, setting the table, foods with interactive questions and fruit/vegetable identification are presented with colorful, simple and inviting illustrations.

Oliver's Vegetables

by Vivian French, Illustrated by Alison Bartlett, Orchard Books, 1995, ISBN 0-531-09462-6

When Oliver goes to visit his grandfather, the only vegetable he will eat is french fries. Soon after his arrival, his experiences in Grandpa's garden result in a whole new world of vegetable tastes for Oliver! The book includes beautiful illustrations.

Potluck

by Anne Shelby, Illustrated by Irene Trivas, Orchard Books, 1991, ISBN 0-531-05919-7

Alpha and Betty plan a potluck and my, what a feast it turns into! All of their friends bring a dish to match their name, corresponding to each letter of the alphabet. The book exemplifies a diversity of children and includes a wide variety of interesting foods such as asparagus soup, kale, peanut-butter pie, quiche, vegetarian stew, yams & yogurt and a zucchini casserole.

The Edible Pyramid: Good Eating Every Day

by Loreen Leedy, Holiday House, 1994, ISBN 0-8234-1126-5

Children will enjoy the whimsical animal characters who manage and patronize "The Edible Pyramid" restaurant. The book is a basic introduction to the Food Guide Pyramid, giving simple information about foods included in each food group and the suggested number of servings to eat each day.

The Vegetable Show

by Laurie Krasney Brown, Little Brown, & Co., 1995, ISBN 0-316-11363-8

A very creative and delightful approach to good nutrition, this book may motivate children to develop their own funny vegetable-based performances. Stars in Brown's book include Wee Peas and Ms. Shelly, Magic by Bud the Spud, Lotta Root the Carrot, Last of the Red Hot Peppers and a finale by the Veggettes. Children will enjoy the vaudeville theme and delightful cut-paper art.

This is the Way We Eat Our Lunch

by Edith Baer, Illustrated by Steve Bjorkman, Scholastic, 1995, ISBN 0-590-46887-1

This simple picture/rhyming book takes children around the United States and then on to other parts of the world to explore what children are eating for lunch. From clam chowder in Massachusetts to sweet potato pie in South Carolina to beans and rice in Ghana, the book illustrates how children around the world nourish their bodies with a wide variety of foods. Included is a map of the world, three recipes and definitions.

Vegetables, Vegetables!

by Fay Robinson, Children's Press, Inc., 1994, ISBN 0-516-06030-9

A picture/word book with colorful photographs of vegetables, this simple book communicates the science concept that vegetables come from the various parts of plants. Different ways to prepare vegetables and how vegetables are grown are also covered.

When I Eat (Preschool–K)

by Mandy Suhr, Carolrhoda Books, 1992, ISBN 0-87614-596-9

This picture book shows food in a simple, colorful manner that preschoolers will enjoy. It explains how people, animals, and plants make use of their food and the proper foods needed for good health.

ALL AGES

Blue Potatoes, Orange Tomatoes

by Rosalind Creasy, Illustrated by Ruth Heller, 1994, Sierra Club Books for Children, ISBN 0-87156-576-5

Kids of all ages will be inspired to start a colorful garden after they finish this book! Creasy gives clear and specific instructions on how to grow an organic rainbow garden. Besides blue potatoes and orange tomatoes, young gardeners will also learn how to grow multi-colored radishes, yellow watermelon and more! Fun and colorful recipes such as "Red, White, and Blue Potato Salad" and "Confetti Bean Salad" are also splashed throughout this delightful book.

Dinosaurs Alive and Well

by Laurie Krasny Brown and Marc Brown, 1990, Little, Brown, & Co., ISBN 0-316-10998-3

If dinosaurs had access to this information, perhaps they would still be alive today! This book is a delightful cartoon book made up of short chapters that will help children develop good health habits. "Eat Up," the chapter on nutrition, gives very clear, accurate advice about the importance of good nutrition and a balanced diet. Other chapters help children to deal with their feelings, take care of themselves, the importance of exercise, friends, hygiene and recovering from illness.

Everybody Bakes Bread
by Norah Dooley, 1996, Carolrhoda Books, ISBN 0-87614-895-X

Building on the success of "Everybody Cooks Rice," Norah Dooley has once again worked a charming story into a lesson about various cultures and the different breads they bake. Delicious recipes from many cultures are included.

Kids Garden! The Anytime, Anyplace Guide to Sowing & Growing Fun
by Avery Hart and Paul Mantell, 1996, Williamson Publishing Co., ISBN 0-913589-90-X

This book has just about everything the young gardener needs to know about the science and art of plants and gardening! Full of solid gardening information and fun, captivating gardening projects, children, teachers and parents will find lots of useful and creative ideas. An outdoor salsa garden, a fast-food salad window box (ready in just three weeks!), and a chapter titled "Munch! Crunch! Grow Your Lunch!" are just a few of the high points in this wonderful book.

The Food Cycle
by David Smith, 1993, Thomson Learning, ISBN 1-56847-093-2

A factual, yet interesting resource book for children who are beginning to learn about nutrition or preparing reports about nutrition and the food cycle. The book includes 13 short chapters on topics such as where foods are grown, food additives, digestion and a healthy diet.

The Kids' Multicultural Cookbook—Food & Fun Around the World
by Deanna F. Cook, 1995, Williamson Publishing Company, ISBN 0-913589-91-8

This is a wonderful way to introduce new tastes and learn interesting facts about various cultures. Deanna Cook has traveled the globe, talking with children and learning about customs and foods. The book includes a marvelous "Let's Get Cooking" introduction with kitchen safety/sanitation basics, and chapters on Asia, Europe, Africa/The Middle East, The Americas and the South Pacific. Recipes are identified according to difficulty. Highly Recommended!

Vegetables
by Susan Wake, 1990, Carolrhoda Books, ISBN 0-87614-390-7

Very factual, this is a great book to begin a unit on plants, gardening or nutrition. Wake discusses vegetables as parts of plants, their nutrition, the historical role of vegetables and the part they play in festivals and celebrations. She includes three step-by-step illustrated recipes (corn fritters, Russian salad, vegetable broth) and instructions on how to "Grow your own peas." A very colorful book with nice photos, it is also a great source for interesting facts about vegetables around the world.

It's Hugh-Man
(and the Foodettes)

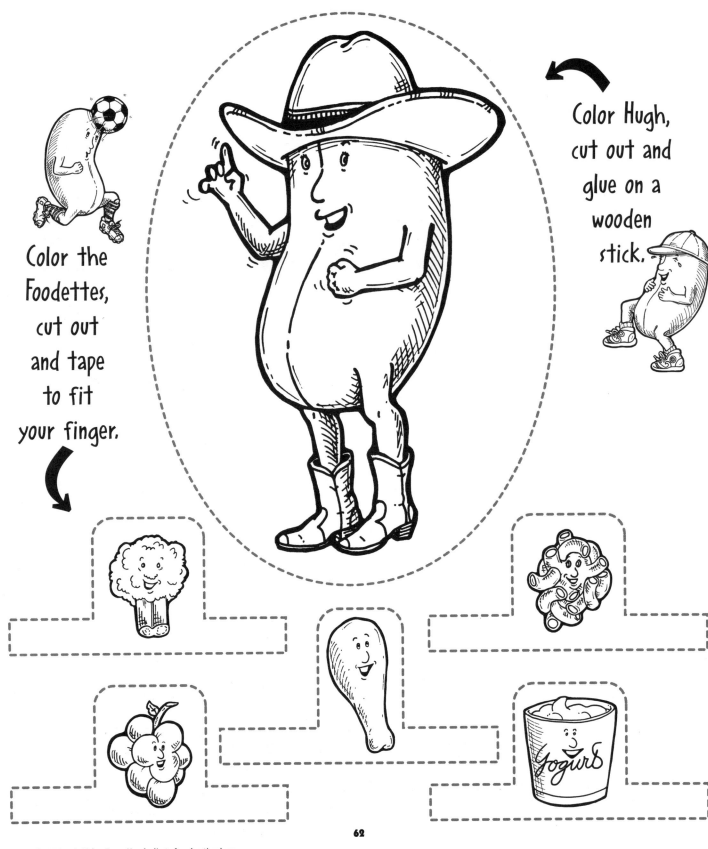

Color the Foodettes, cut out and tape to fit your finger.

Color Hugh, cut out and glue on a wooden stick.

62

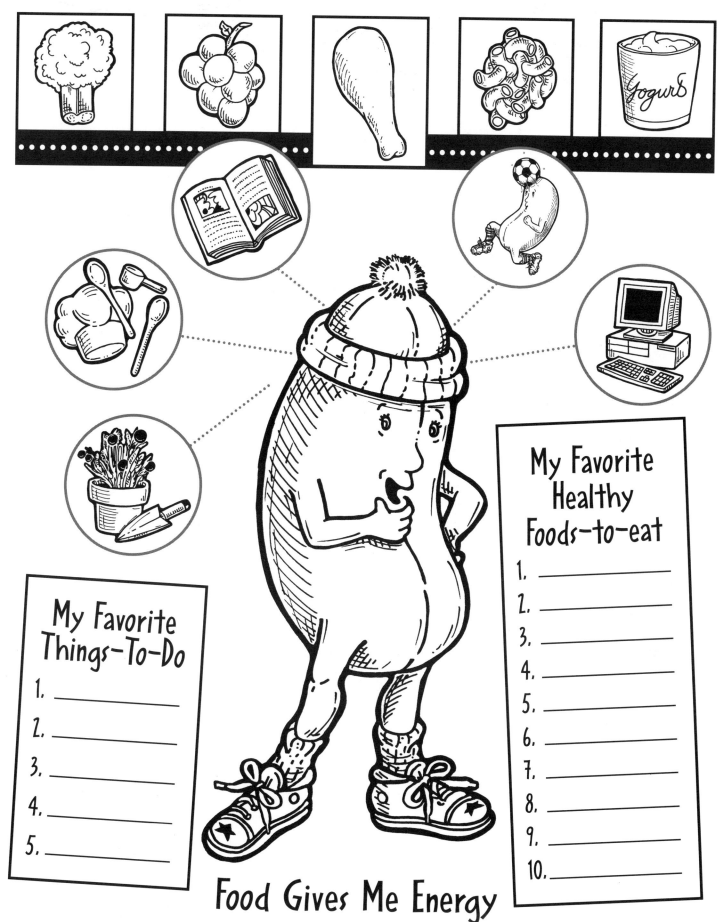

My Favorite Healthy Foods-to-eat

1. _____
2. _____
3. _____
4. _____
5. _____
6. _____
7. _____
8. _____
9. _____
10. _____

My Favorite Things-To-Do

1. _____
2. _____
3. _____
4. _____
5. _____

Food Gives Me Energy
So I Can Do...MY FAVORITE THINGS!...How About You?

ORDER FORM

HOW TO TEACH NUTRITION TO KIDS: An integrated, creative approach
to nutrition education for children ages 6–10 (ISBN 0-9647970-3-8)
_____ copies at $18.00 per copy $ _____

LEADER/ACTIVITY GUIDE: A companion to *How to Teach Nutrition
to Kids*. (ISBN 0-9647970-6-2)
_____ copies at $11.95 per copy $ _____

Shipping and Handling
$2.50 per book for 1st book; $1.00 for each additional book $ _____

TOTAL ENCLOSED $ _____

Name/Affiliation _____

Address _____

City _____ State _____ Zip _____

Telephone _____ Fax _____ Email _____

MasterCard/VISA # _____ Exp. Date _____

Authorized Signature _____

Send payment to: 24 CARROT PRESS, P.O. Box 23546, Tigard, OR 97281-3546; Phone/Fax: 1-800-291-6098;
Email: eversc@teleport.com *Quantity Discounts Available—Call for Rates.*

HOW TO TEACH NUTRITION TO KIDS: An integrated, creative approach
to nutrition education for children ages 6–10 (ISBN 0-9647970-3-8)
_____ copies at $18.00 per copy $ _____

LEADER/ACTIVITY GUIDE: A companion to *How to Teach Nutrition
to Kids*. (ISBN 0-9647970-6-2)
_____ copies at $11.95 per copy $ _____

Shipping and Handling
$2.50 per book for 1st book; $1.00 for each additional book $ _____

TOTAL ENCLOSED $ _____

Name/Affiliation _____

Address _____

City _____ State _____ Zip _____

Telephone _____ Fax _____ Email _____

MasterCard/VISA # _____ Exp. Date _____

Authorized Signature _____

Send payment to: 24 CARROT PRESS, P.O. Box 23546, Tigard, OR 97281-3546; Phone/Fax: 1-800-291-6098;
Email: eversc@teleport.com *Quantity Discounts Available—Call for Rates.*